ISRAEL

REPRODUCTION AND ABORTION: LAW AND POLICY

Law Library of Congress

ISBN-10   1511677996

ISBN-13   978-1511677998

LAW LIBRARY OF CONGRESS

ISRAEL

REPRODUCTION AND ABORTION: LAW AND POLICY

TABLE OF CONTENTS

LAW LIBRARY OF CONGRESS

ISRAEL

REPRODUCTION AND ABORTION: LAW AND POLICY

Executive Summary

Israel has maintained a pro-natalist policy with regard to reproductive care. The State provides health care along the continuum from family planning services through childbirth. Much of reproductive care is funded by the government and through Health Funds. This report analyzes various factors that have impacted Israel's approach to reproductive care and discusses the governing law as well as the types and amounts of government funding that are allocated for reproductive care.

Israel's reproductive care policy appears to reflect Jewish religious, cultural, and social norms regarding fertility. Parenthood is considered a basic human right based on biblical and other Jewish religious sources. The personal desire for parenthood, and specifically motherhood, has been engrained in Jewish culture and has been strengthened by the historical persecution of Jews in the Diaspora and particularly by the genocide perpetrated against Jews in the Holocaust. The continuing loss of life in Arab-Israeli wars and terrorist acts, combined with constant threats to the State's existence by hostile powers in the region, have also been linked to Israelis' attitudes regarding procreation.

Israel's pro-natalist approach is supported by legislation regulating in vitro fertilization (IVF), ova extraction, the use of semen in IVF fertilization, ova donation and allocation, and surrogacy agreements. The regulation of assisted reproductive technology (ART) in Israel appears to support reproductive choice while respecting certain religious and cultural considerations.

A person's right to procreate has been recognized in Supreme Court rulings, especially in the leading case of Nachmani v. Nachmani, where the Court held that in the special circumstances of that case the right of a woman to motherhood was superior to her husband's right not to be a father.

The recognition of the importance of parenthood and the superior right to motherhood, however, has not resulted in recognition of a woman's full autonomy over her reproductive status. By law, a woman does not have a general right to choose to terminate her pregnancy. An interruption of pregnancy may be permitted under certain circumstances by special committees for the interruption of pregnancies established by hospitals or the Ministry of Health. Such circumstances include the age of the woman; the pregnancy deriving from rape, incest, or an out-of-wedlock relationship; and fetal disabilities and physical or mental danger to the *mother posed by continuation of the pregnancy. In spite of these restrictions, in reality, abortions are performed in Israel, with and without authorization. The penal provision that prohibits unauthorized abortions does not appear ever to have been enforced.*

The lack of interest in prosecution reflects the limited scope of the abortion debate in Israel. It has been reported that over 98% of all requests for abortions to the committees have been approved and that the rate of abortions has generally declined in recent years. In addition to funding legally authorized abortions, the State funds the provision of family planning information and subsidizes contraceptives.

In spite of the general low level of interest in this topic, an increased awareness of competing views on abortions has been sparked with the introduction of a bill in 2009 designed to repeal the legal requirement for a committees' approval for abortions. Religious leaders and their representatives in the Knesset have recently expressed objections to abortion procedures based on religious grounds. A bill calling for prohibiting abortions under any circumstances following the twenty-second week of pregnancy has been twice defeated, most recently in November 2011.

There are several Israeli as well as American PACs and NGOs with opposite agendas on reproductive policy in Israel. They, however, do not appear to have any significant impact on reproductive policy in Israel.

I. Introduction

Israel has one of the highest birth and fertility rates among industrialized countries.[1] Although the average age of women giving birth for the first time has consistently increased in the past ten years, modern technologies such as in vitro fertilization (IVF) and the use of assisted reproductive technology (ART), along with a pro-natalist state policy fully or partially subsidizing such treatments, have made it possible for an increased number of women, including unmarried or infertile women and those wishing to delay procreation to facilitate career development, to give birth.

Israel's state policy regarding reproductive rights has been linked to its strong Jewish religious tradition, Jewish quest for survival, "the dreadful memory of the Holocaust, the permanent loss of life in terrorist attacks and military battles, the demographic concern caused by competition with surrounding Arab nations, and the strong cultural perception of raising a family as a patriotic endeavor."[2]

The State's pro-natalist policy, however, has not resulted in the prevention of abortions. Under the Penal Law, interruption of a pregnancy is a criminal offense if conducted in the absence of an approval as regulated by law. In reality, the overwhelming majority of requests for legal abortions are approved. Moreover, to date there have been no known cases where a doctor

---

[1] Daniel Sperling, *Commanding the "Be Fruitful and Multiply" Directive: Reproductive Ethics, Law, and Policy in Israel*, 19 CAMBRIDGE Q. OF HEALTHCARE ETHICS 363-71 (2010).

[2] *Id.*

was indicted for the unauthorized interruption of a pregnancy in violation of the penal law, as discussed below.

This report describes Israel's specific policies and law on reproductive technologies and abortions and discusses their social, religious, and political context.

II. Current Laws and Regulations Regarding Reproductive Rights

A. Prenatal Care Insurance Coverage

Israel maintains a system of national health care. In accordance with the National Health Insurance Law, 5754-1994,[3] Israeli residents are entitled to medical services that are provided by Health Funds that are approved by the Ministry of Health. The Health Funds must provide services that are included in "a basket of basic health services," which includes specific reproductive health services and products.[4] The scope of technologies and medications to be included in the basket of basic health services, within the budget allocation, is determined on a yearly basis by a public committee appointed for that purpose by the Minister of Health.[5]

Insured patients are entitled to be provided with oral contraceptives.[6] In addition, they are entitled to prenatal care; interruption of pregnancy for medical reasons, as well as for non-medical reasons in the case of girls under nineteen years of age; fetal organ system exams; *epidurals during birth*; exams for identification of fetal disabilities, including amniocentesis, etc.[7]

Israeli residents are also entitled to genetic counseling, including blood tests and genetic evaluation. Such evaluation is provided to carriers of genetic or chromosomal interference or of especially severe genetic diseases, to couples with a high probability of giving birth to a child with especially serious chromosomal disabilities, and to women who have undergone repeated miscarriages. Entitlement to prenatal genetic evaluation is limited to two pregnancies resulting in birth. Israeli women are also permitted to undergo extraction of ova for freezing for future implantation for any reason. The procedure and the freezing of the ova are fully covered when done for medical reasons, and the maximum amount of coverage for other reasons is to be determined by the Ministry of Health.[8]

---

[3] National Health Insurance Law, 5754-1994, SEFER HA-HUKIM [SH] [BOOK OF LAWS, Official Gazette] , p. 156, *as amended*.

[4] *Id.* § 7 & 2d Supp., *as amended*, *available at* http://www.nevo.co.il (legal database in Hebrew; last visited Feb. 1, 2012).

[5] Memorandum issued by the Knesset Information and Research Center (KIRC) (Mar. 22, 2011) (on file with author).

[6] Public Health Insurance Decree (Pharmaceuticals in the Health Services Basket) 5755-1995, KOVETZ HATAKANOT [KT] [SUBSIDIARY REGULATIONS] No. 5662, p. 749.

[7] National Health Insurance Law, 5754-1994, 2d Supp., § 7.

[8] *Id.* §§ 21-22.

In 2010 the Ministry of Health appointed a special public committee to review and propose various reproductive services that had not been not regulated by law. The committee, titled "the Public Committee for the Legislative Evaluation of Fertility and Birth in Israel" (the Committee), solicited public comments and information to be received by February 2, 2011.[9] By February 3, 2012, the date of completion of this report, the Committee's recommendations had not yet been published.

Among the subjects expected to be reviewed by the Committee are accessibility of fertility technologies by segments of the population, by couples or singles, depending on their family situation; the use of advanced reproductive technologies to prevent genetically transmitted disease; the status of fertility treatments that were conducted abroad, including those commencing outside of Israel but concluding in Israel; and the determination of parental status regarding children born by using different fertility technologies.[10]

B. In Vitro Fertilization (IVF) and Ova Extraction for Personal Use

Public Health (In Vitro Fertilization) Regulations 5747-1987 were issued by the Minister of Health in April 1987.[11] The regulations require that any extraction, fertilization, or implantation of ova from or in a woman's body must be done in a hospital department that has officially been accredited in the official gazette for performing activities related to IVF (hereafter IVF accredited department).[12] The regulations establish specific requirements for the implantation of ova that were extracted and fertilized outside of Israel in a woman in Israel.[13]

1. *Ova Extraction*

The regulations limit the extraction of ova to women undergoing fertility treatments and those interested in preserving their fertility who are thirty to forty-one years old, as long as they undergo not more than four extractions and the number of ova extracted is fewer than twenty.[14]

A directive issued by the Ministry of Health in January 2011 pursuant to the above regulations specifies that the extraction procedure may include hormonal treatments for three to four weeks, extractions under full anesthesia, and the freezing of ova for future implantation in a woman of fifty-four years or younger.[15] Hospitals that are licensed to conduct these procedures may charge patients up to specific amounts that are determined by the Ministry of Health. When

---

[9] The Public Committee for the Legislative Evaluation of Fertility and Birth in Israel, Israel's Ministry of Health, http://www.old.health.gov.il/pages/default.asp?maincat=1&catid=6&pageid=5171 (last visited Jan. 30, 2012).

[10] *Id.*

[11] Public Health (In Vitro Fertilization) Regulations 5747-1987, KT No. 5035, p. 987.

[12] *Id.* § 2.

[13] *Id.* § 2A.

[14] *Id.* § 4.

[15] Freezing of Ova for Preservation of a Woman's Fertility, Directive No. 1/2001, MINISTRY OF HEALTH (Jan. 9, 2011), http://www.health.gov.il/hozer/mr01_2011.pdf.

the freezing of ova is necessitated by a medical reason specified by the directive, however, it is fully covered by Israeli health funds, based on their inclusion in the basket of basic health services, as determined by the Ministry of Health.[16]

2. *Use of Semen for In Vitro Fertilization*

The regulations set special conditions for the use of semen for in vitro fertilization. Ova extracted from a married woman will not be fertilized with the semen of a donor or semen received from the donors' bank unless both the donor of the ova and her husband consent to the implant in advance and in writing.[17] Similarly, ova of a donor will not be fertilized with the semen of the husband of the woman in which they will be implanted after fertilization in the absence of such consent.[18]

The regulations permit the implantation of fertilized ova in single women subject to the following conditions:

- The ova are hers and a report by a social worker of the IVF accredited department supports her request;

- The fertilized ova's owner was widowed prior to the implantation, as long as the fertilized ova will not be implanted in her during the first year following the extraction and fertilization of the ova and the implantation is supported by a report as detailed above; or

- The woman in whom implantation is planned is a divorcee whose ova were fertilized with her husband's semen prior to the divorce, only after receipt of the husband's consent.[19]

The regulations generally prohibit the implantation of ova of deceased spouses and implantation in relatives of ova donors in the absence of predetermined circumstances.[20] They further require informed consent from each spouse for any IVF activities and the husband's consent for any IVF activity of a married woman.[21] The regulations prohibit the disclosure of identifying information regarding ova or semen donors.[22]

---

[16] Dan Even, *Freezing of Ova Permitted for Women (in Israel) Also for Career Considerations*, HAARETZ ONLINE (FEB. 1, 2012), http://www.haaretz.co.il/hasite/spages/1210255.html (in Hebrew).

[17] Public Health (In Vitro Fertilization) Regulations 5747-1987, § 6, KT No. 5035, p. 987.

[18] *Id.* § 7.

[19] *Id.* § 8.

[20] *Id.* §§ 10, 12.

[21] *Id.* § 14.

[22] *Id.* § 15

C. Ova Donation

1. *General Principles*

The Knesset passed the Ova Donation Law, 5770-2010,[23] on June 13, 2010. The law declares that its objective is

> [t]o regulate donation of ova for the purpose of birth, while ensuring the dignity, rights and health of the donor and the recipient, as well as regulating the use of ova for research purposes, and all the while preserving the status of women.[24]

According to the law, when a treating physician has concluded that a patient who is an Israeli resident eighteen to fifty-three years of age is incapable of getting pregnant from ova produced by her body because of a medical problem or has another medical problem that justifies use of the ova of another woman for the birth of a child, including by implant in a surrogate mother, he will notify the patient that she may submit a petition for ova donation.[25] The law defines a "treating physician" as a holder of the title of specialist in obstetrics and gynecology employed in an IVF accredited department who has been trained in the IVF unit.[26]

The law provides that a child born as a consequence of ova donation will be considered the child of the ova recipient.[27] The donation severs any relationship of the donor and her relatives to the child.[28]

The law restricts the extraction and donation of ova exclusively for the purpose of the birth of a child.[29] Under certain conditions, however, ova that were extracted for this purpose may be used for research.[30] The law regulates the export of ova outside of Israel and the provision of medical treatment in donors and recipients for the performance of surrogacy motherhood contracts.[31] The law also prohibits trade in ova[32] and requires full confidentiality for any information received in the course of any work related to IVF treatment.[33] The law further provides for various penalties for violations of its provisions.[34]

---

[23] Ova Donation Law, 5770-2010, SH No. 2242, p. 520.

[24] *Id.* § 1 (translated by the author, R.L.).

[25] *Id.* § 11.

[26] *Id.*

[27] *Id.* § 42(a).

[28] *Id.* § 42(c).

[29] *Id.* § 3.

[30] *Id.* §§ 27-29.

[31] *Id.* §§ 5-7.

[32] *Id.* §§ 8-10.

[33] *Id.* § 38.

[34] *Id.* § 41.

2. *Conditions for Extraction*

The extraction of ova from a donor requires the written approval of a special committee representing both genders that is appointed for each particular case by the hospital manager (hereafter the "approval committee") and composed of the following members:

- A specialist physician who heads a hospital department that does not deal with obstetrics, gynecology, or IVF, who heads the committee;

- A specialist in obstetrics and gynecology who has experience in IVF and is not the treating physician;

- A clinical psychologist;

- A social worker;

- An attorney; and

- A public representative or a religious official, according to the donor's request, who, to the extent possible, belongs to her religious, social, or cultural group.[35]

A request to donate ova must be submitted to the approval committee by the donor after she has been provided with information in writing, in a language she understands, of the following:

- The possible direct and indirect risks related to extraction of ova;

- The details to be kept in a data bank and registry, and the conditions of their release;

- Her rights and prohibitions under the law;

- Her rights to designate ova for implant, freezing for her future use, research, or disposal, and to later change her designation;

- The status of the newborn; and

- The circumstances in which approval of a special National Exceptions Committee (hereafter NEC) is required.[36]

Upon submitting her request, the donor will undergo both medical and psychological tests to examine her suitability to donate ova in accordance with the law.[37]

The approval committee may approve the request after having verified that the donor

- is an Israeli resident twenty-one to thirty-four years old;

---

[35] *Id.* § 12(b).

[36] *Id.* § 12(d). *See* discussion of the NEC, page 9, *infra*.

[37] *Id.* § 12(e).

- has legal capacity, is capable of taking care of her livelihood needs, and is not detained or under arrest;

- signed a consent form before the approval committee;

- granted her consent with a clear mind and free will and not due to family, social, economic, or other pressure; and,

- in cases where she designated her ova to a specific recipient ahead of the extraction, granted her consent without consideration of financial or any other compensation.[38]

3. *Conditions for Ova Allocation and Implantation*

The allocation of ova extracted from a donor and their implantation in a recipient or in a surrogate in accordance with the Surrogacy Motherhood Agreement Law requires the approval of the head of an IVF accredited department or his designee.[39] This approval authority is strictly regulated. For example, except for semen from the semen bank, implantation will not be approved in the absence of the semen donor's written consent ahead of time for one or more implantations and the recordation of his personal data in both a data bank and a newborn registry, in accordance with the law.[40]

The law further requires a showing of the following as a precondition for approval of implantation:

- The recipient is an Israeli resident eighteen to fifty-three years old;

- The treating physician has determined that the recipient is incapable, because of a medical problem, of being impregnated or has a different medical problem that justifies the use of another woman's ova for giving birth;[41]

- The head of the IVF accredited department or his deputy (hereafter the "responsible physician") has received confirmation from the Ministry of Health databank for IVF relevant information that the donor belongs to the same religion of the recipient and is not related to her, is not related to the designated genetic father, and is not married; and

- If the ova are extracted from a woman who is married or who does not belong to the religion of the recipient, the responsible physician should inform the recipient and her spouse, as appropriate, of this information and accept their written consent to obtain ova from the donor.[42]

---

[38] *Id.* § 12(f).

[39] *Id.* § 13(a).

[40] *Id.* § 13(d).

[41] The law defines a "treating physician" as a physician who holds the title of specialist in obstetrics and gynecology in an accredited department, who has undergone training in the IVF department and has been assigned by the department head to be a treating physician under the Ova Donation Law. *Id.* § 2.

[42] *Id.* § 13(e).

The Law strictly regulates the procedures for designation and documentation of ova extraction and use and requires that the donor be informed of the number of ova extracted from her body and their quality prior to signing a consent form for the ova designated for implantation, freezing for her future use, research, or destruction.[43]   The number of ova designated by a donor for freezing for future use by her or for research, however, must not exceed 20% of the number of ova extracted from her body or two ova, whichever is less.[44]

4. *Exceptions*

The law requires preapproval by the National Exceptions Committee (NEC) for the extraction, designation, or implantation from a donor who predesignates her ova to a specific recipient or a donor who is married or does not belong to the recipient's religion, and it similarly requires preapproval to export ova outside of Israel.[45]   The NEC is composed of several members, appointed by the Minister of Health, who represent both genders, including a specialist who previously served as the head of a gynecological, obstetrics, or fertility department in a hospital; an additional specialist physician; a psychologist; a social worker; and an attorney; a religious official of both the donor's and the recipient's religion, or of both religions when they differ.[46]

In approving requests under one of the IVF exceptions, the NEC must consider both religious and social grounds that justify predesignation of ova to specific recipients. Accordingly, the NEC may approve a request by a donor to designate ova implantation in a specific recipient who is a relative of the donor if the donation is justified by religious considerations; similarly, the NEC may authorize a donor's request to designate her ova to be implanted in a recipient who is not her relative based on relevant religious or social considerations.[47]

The law further specifies circumstances where the NEC may recognize exceptions to the general prohibition against ova donations by married donors. Such exceptions may be approved when there are religious reasons for such donations and when such donations are necessary because of a shortage in ova donations from unmarried donors.[48]

The NEC is also authorized to approve the extraction and implantation of ova in a recipient who is not of the donor's religious affiliation because the religion of the recipient prohibits her from obtaining a donation from a member of her faith or because there are not enough available ova from members of her religious community.[49]

---

[43] *Id.* §§ 16-19.

[44] *Id.* § 16(a), (b), (c).

[45] *Id.* § 20(a).

[46] *Id.* § 20(b).

[47] *Id.* § 22(a).

[48] *Id.* § 22(b).

[49] *Id.* § 22(c).

The NEC is similarly authorized to approve the donation of ova to a recipient for implantation outside of Israel if it finds that there is justification for such an action.[50]

5. *Compensation for Donors*

The State reimburses the donor for undergoing extraction of ova for the purpose of implantation in an amount established by the Minister of Health, with the consent of the Minister of the Treasury and the approval of the Knesset Committee for Labor, Welfare and Health. The State also reimburses a donor who is a patient half of that amount for her consent to allocate extra ova for implantation.[51] The money paid to donors is partially derived from the fee paid by applicants requesting approval for ova implantation.[52]

D. Surrogate Motherhood

On March 17, 1996, the Knesset passed the Agreements for the Carriage of Fetuses (Approval of Agreement and Status of the New Born) Law, 5756-1996[53] (hereafter the "Surrogacy Agreements Law").

1. *Surrogacy Agreements*

The implantation of fertilized ova for the purpose of conception by a surrogate mother in order to transfer the child that will be born to the designated parents requires that the following conditions are met:[54]

- A written agreement between the surrogate mother and the designated parents has been approved by the approval committee;

- The parties to the agreement are eighteen years old or older and are Israeli residents;

- The surrogate mother

  --is unmarried (except that the approval committee may approve a surrogate who is married if it is convinced that the designated parents could not, after reasonable effort, engage in a surrogacy agreement with a surrogate who is single) and

  --is not a relative of any of the designated parents;

- The semen used for the IVF is of the designated father and the ova is not of the surrogate;

---

[50] *Id.* § 22(d).

[51] *Id.* § 43.

[52] *Id.* § 47.

[53] Agreements for the Carriage of Fetuses (Approval of Agreement and Status of the Newborn) Law, 5756-1996 (hereafter "Surrogacy Agreements Law"), SH No. 1577, p. 176.

[54] *Id.* § 2.

- The surrogate belongs to the same religion as the designated mother, but if all parties to the agreement are not Jewish the committee may deviate from this requirement in accordance with an opinion of a religious official who is a member of the committee.

2. *The Approval Committee*

The Surrogacy Agreements Law requires surrogacy agreements to be approved by a committee to be appointed by the Minister of Health. The Committee must include

- two doctors with the title of specialist in obstetrics and gynecology;
- a doctor with the title of specialist in internal medicine;
- a clinical psychologist;
- a social worker;
- a public representative who is a lawyer; and
- a religious official of the religion of the parties to the surrogacy agreement.[55]

3. *Conditions for Approval of Surrogacy Agreements*

The request for approval should include the following:

- A proposal for an agreement for surrogacy;
- A medical opinion regarding the inability of the designated mother to become pregnant and carry the pregnancy or stating that a pregnancy may significantly endanger her health;
- A medical and a psychological opinion regarding the suitability of all parties to the procedure;
- Confirmation by a psychologist or a social worker that the designated parents have received a suitable professional consultation, including regarding other parenthood options; and
- If the parties entered a surrogacy agreement through an intermediary for a fee, information regarding the intermediary contract and the identity of the intermediary must also be provided to the approval committee.[56]

The approval committee may request to see additional materials and summon other persons as it sees fit. After evaluating all the documents and testimony, the committee may approve the request if it is convinced that the following conditions have been met:

---

[55] *Id.* § 3.

[56] *Id.* § 4.

- All parties entered the surrogacy agreement voluntarily and with an understanding of its meaning and consequences;

- No danger to the health of the surrogate or the newborn appears to exist; and

- The surrogacy agreements did not include conditions that could harm or disadvantage the rights of the newborn or any of the parties.

Following approval, the surrogacy agreement must be signed in the presence of the committee. Any change in the agreement must be approved by the committee. The committee is further authorized to reevaluate its approval if any substantial change in the facts, circumstances, or conditions that served as a basis for its approval occurs, as long as the fertilized ova has not yet been implanted in the surrogate mother in accordance with the Surrogacy Agreements Law.[57]

III. Regulation of Abortion and Penalties for Illegal Abortions

The Penal Law, 5737-1977,[58] as amended, imposes a penalty of a five-year imprisonment or a fine on "[a]ny person who knowingly interrupts a woman's pregnancy, either by medical treatment or in any other manner …."[59] A woman who undergoes an unlawful abortion, however, does not bear any criminal liability.[60]

This provision notwithstanding, a search for penalties imposed on offenders who violated section 313 has not revealed any case in which a physician was prosecuted for performing an abortion. Cases where offenders were convicted for committing the offense of interruption of pregnancy are relatively rare and usually involve violent, criminal offenses. In 2001, for example, the Supreme Court confirmed the conviction of a married physician who solicited three persons to interrupt the pregnancy of his lover by assaulting her.[61]

A. Exemptions from Criminal Liability

The Law exempts from criminal liability any gynecologist who interrupted a woman's pregnancy at a recognized medical institution following an approval by that institution's Committee for Interruption of Pregnancies.[62]

The Law further exempts a qualified physician from criminal liability for interruption of pregnancy if the interruption was urgently required in order to save the life of the woman or prevent her from incurring a serious uncorrectable harm. A qualified physician is similarly

---

[57] *Id.* § 5.

[58] Penal Law, 5737-1977, LAWS OF THE STATE OF ISRAEL [LSI] (Authorized Translation from the Hebrew Prepared at the Ministry of Justice) (Special Volume) (1977), *as amended.*

[59] *Id.* § 313.

[60] *Id.* § 320.

[61] *See, e.g.,* CA 1655/00 State of Israel v. Fuad Musa (Nov. 12, 2001), *available at* the Nevo Legal Database (by subscription).

[62] Penal Law, 5737-1977, § 314.

exempted from liability if the interruption occurred in the course of providing a different medical treatment in the woman's body, when the pregnancy was not previously known to the physician and the interruption was necessary for that medical treatment. The exemption under these conditions requires a detailed written notification within five days following the procedure.[63]

B. The Committee for Interruption of Pregnancies

1. *Composition*

The Committee for Interruption of Pregnancies (CIP) is designated by the manager of a hospital registered under the Public Health Ordinance 1940,[64] as amended, or, in the case of any other recognized medical institution, by the Minister of Health. The committee must consist of at least one woman and include

- a qualified medical practitioner holding the title of specialist in obstetrics and gynecology;
- another qualified medical practitioner practicing obstetrics and gynecology, internal medicine, psychiatry, family medicine, or public health; and
- a registered social worker.[65]

2. *Grounds for Approval of Abortions*

In accordance with the Penal Law, the committee may, after having received the woman's informed consent, grant permission for interruption of her pregnancy if it has determined that termination is justified based on one of the following reasons:

- The woman is under seventeen or over forty years old;
- The pregnancy derives from a relationship that is prohibited under the penal law, is incestuous, or is out of wedlock;
- The fetus may have a physical or mental disability; or
- Continuation of the pregnancy may endanger the woman's life or cause her physical or mental harm.[66]

A fifth condition—namely, an "economic clause"—was repealed on January 3, 1980.[67] That provision previously authorized the CIP to approve an abortion if "[c]ontinuation of the

---

[63] *Id.* § 317.

[64] Public Health Ordinance 1940, ITON RISHMI (the Official Gazette during the tenure of the Provisional Council of State) No. 1065, 1st App., pp. 191, 239a, *as amended* (full text reflecting all amendments *available at* the NEVO LEGAL DATABASE http://www.nevo.co.il (by subscription)).

[65] Penal Law, 5737-1977, § 315, LSI (Special Volume) (1977), *as amended.*

[66] *Id.* § 316(a).

[67] *Id.*

pregnancy might cause a serious harm to the woman or her children, based on the harsh family or social conditions of the woman and her environment."[68]

The law requires the woman to provide informed consent for interruption of her pregnancy in writing after being informed of the physical and mental risks associated with the interruption of pregnancy.[69] The law clearly states that consent by a minor does not require approval by her parents or guardians.[70] Furthermore, a woman's request cannot be rejected unless she was given an opportunity to appear before the committee and explain her reasons.[71] Approval of a request for interruption of pregnancy by the committee does not bind any gynecologist if performing an abortion is against his conscience or medical opinion.[72]

IV. Political Context to the Abortion Debate in Israel

A. Statistical Data

Although Israeli law imposes strict limitations on abortions, in practice 98.5% of all requests for abortions to the committees were approved in 2009, and 98.7% in 2010.[73] According to a press release issued by the Central Bureau of Statistics on September 20, 2011, the percentage of abortions performed in Israel has decreased from 15.2 of any 100 known pregnancies in 1988 to 11.0 in 2009.[74] Between 2007 and 2009, the percentage of abortions known to have been performed in Israel was lower than that in Western Europe. As compared with the United States, the United Kingdom, and Canada, the abortion rate from 2006–2010 was similarly much lower.[75]

Additional information further indicates that 13.3% of the total applications for approval of interruption of pregnancy in Israel were submitted by women younger than nineteen years of age, 51.4% involved a pregnancy out of wedlock, and 19.1% a pregnancy involving fetal physiological or mental defect.[76]

---

[68] *See* the Penal Law 5737-1977, § 316(5), repealed by Amendment No. 8, SH No. 954, p. 40, *available at* the NEVO LEGAL DATABASE http://www.nevo.co.il (by subscription).

[69] *Id.* § 316(b).

[70] *Id.*

[71] *Id.* § 316(c).

[72] *Id.* § 318.

[73] Press Release, State of Israel Central Bureau of Statistics, Application for Pregnancy Termination in 2009, and Temporary Data 2010 (Sept. 20, 2011), http://www.cbs.gov.il/reader/newhodaot/hodaa_template.html?hodaa=201105237.

[74] *Id.* at 4.

[75] *Id.* at 9.

[76] *Id.* at 1, 6-8; For additional detailed information *see Interruption of Pregnancy under the Law, 1990-2010,* MINISTRY OF HEALTH (Nov. 2011), http://www.health.gov.il/PublicationsFiles/preg1990_2010.pdf.

B. State Policy

The State supports family planning and subsidizes both contraceptives and abortions. Abortions involving teens nineteen years of age or younger are fully funded.[77] Abortions related to fetal defects, rape, or incest are similarly funded; abortions for out-of-wedlock pregnancies, however, are only partially subsidized.[78]

In January 2011, when an earlier study on Israel's reproductive policies was conducted by this author, detailed information on interruption of pregnancy was available on the State of Israel, Ministry of Health website. Israel's Ministry of Health website featured a brochure that provided guidance to pregnant teens. This brochure is no longer directly available on the Ministry's website, but was archived.[79]

The brochure emphasizes the teen's right to choose and clarifies that the consent of the teen's partner or parent is not necessary for interruption of pregnancy.[80] Highlighted in the brochure (in special paragraphs in the color pink) were statements such as the following:

> Remember:
> 1. This is your body! Nobody can decide for you and force you to give birth or undergo an abortion.
> 2. Nobody can be 100% sure regarding the "perfect" decision . . ..[81]

> Remember:
> Interruption of pregnancy is not "a contraceptive."[82]

The Ministry of Health brochure provided that the teen was guaranteed complete confidentiality except in cases where disclosure was necessary to protect her from harm or abuse by a relative or a guardian.

The tone of the brochure was supportive and discussed the teen's possible feelings regarding the pregnancy while undergoing an abortion, stating, for example:

> During the interruption of pregnancy, to relieve tension, it is recommended to think and imagine positive adventures:
>   • A walk along the beach or lying down on the grass

---

[77] Expansion of Eligibility for Interruption of Pregnancy for Teens under Nineteen Years of Age, Directive No. 38/2008, MINISTRY OF HEALTH (Sept. 21, 2008), http://www.health.gov.il/hozer/mr38_2008.pdf.

[78] Mital Yasor Beit-Or, *Expensive Abortion: the Price was Increased from 1,400 to 2,200 Shekels*, YNET (Aug. 8, 2010), http://www.ynet.co.il/articles/0,7340,L-3931800,00.html (in Hebrew); for further information on funding of abortion *see* Government Funding for Reproductive Care, section VII, below.

[79] *Information to Teen Girls in an Unplanned Pregnancy*, STATE OF ISRAEL MINISTRY OF HEALTH, http://www.old.health.gov.il/download/pages/preg010210.pdf (last visited Feb. 3, 2012).

[80] *Id*. at 8-9.

[81] *Id*. at 5.

[82] *Id*. at 10.

- A familiar place in which you feel safe
- Travel and finding a new place where you have never been
- Beloved and significant people in your life.[83]

The last portion of the brochure discusses contraceptives and recommends that following the abortion the teen should consider the use of contraceptives to avoid additional pregnancy and sexually transmitted diseases. As throughout the brochure, there was an emphasis on the right of the teen to make choices regarding her pregnancy, as well as regarding whether or not to engage in sexual relations.[84]

C. Political Debate on Abortion and Its Origins

The debate regarding the legality and the appropriateness of abortions in Israel is limited in scope as compared to the debate in the United States. Generally, Jewish Orthodox organizations and political parties, which compose a relative minority in the Israeli public and political sphere, tend to oppose abortions for *Halakhik* (Jewish law) reasons.[85] Leftist parties, on the other hand, have shown interest in removing any restrictions on access to abortions. The majority of Israelis, however, reportedly have not expressed strong positions on this issue.[86]

The introduction of a bill in June 2009 that proposed to void the CIPs in Israel allegedly sparked a political debate on abortions. The bill was introduced by two Knesset Members of the centrist *Kadima* party as well as one of the leftist *Meretz* and communist *Hadash* parties.[87] According to the bill's explanatory notes, the existing abortion procedures under Israeli law are "paternalistic, in that they do not provide the woman with freedom of choice and do not enable her to take responsibility for her choice."[88] The explanatory notes further provide that the specific grounds that are required as a basis for approval of requests for abortions in Israel mean that "the mere wish of a woman to terminate a pregnancy is not a sufficient reason for the Committee's approval."[89]

According to explanatory notes to the bill, the lack of enforcement and the existence of the CIPs have created a disparity between women of means who use private abortion clinics to undergo unauthorized abortions and those of lesser means who must get the CIPs' approval in order to get health insurance coverage. The bill's explanatory notes therefore conclude by

---

[83] *Id.* § 19.

[84] *Id.* § 20.

[85] Jewish law, however, permits abortions under some circumstances, including when the pregnancy threatens the life of the mother. *See, e.g.*, Daniel Eisenberg, Abortion and Halacha, JEWISH VIRTUAL LIBRARY, http://www.jewishvirtuallibrary.org/jsource/Judaism/abortion.html (last visited Feb. 2. 2012).

[86] Yael Hashiloni-Dolev, *Let's Abort Quietly*, YNET (Oct. 30, 2009), http://www.ynet.co.il/articles/0,7340, L-3796232,00.html (in Hebrew).

[87] Voiding the Pregnancies Committee (Amendment) 5769-2009, THE KNESSET WEBSITE, http://www.knesset.gov.il/privatelaw/data/18/1382.rtf (last visited Feb. 1, 2012).

[88] *Id.*

[89] *Id.*

stating that the abortion law is contrary to personal liberties and proposes nullifying the requirement for the CIPs' approval.[90] Knesset Member Nitzan Horowitz, who coauthored the 2009 bill, submitted an additional bill in October 2010, similarly calling for abolition of the CIPs for the same reasons.[91]

In an article published in October 2009, an Israeli scholar warned against rising tensions regarding abortions in Israel in connection with the 2009 bill. The author, Dr. Yael Hashiloni-Dolev, suggested that as compared with the United States, Germany, and Ireland, abortions have never been the subject of a serious public debate in Israel. The only time the abortion issue has been mentioned in Israeli politics is in connection with demands made by *Haredi* (ultra-Orthodox) parties as one of their preconditions for joining coalition agreements. This relates to the repeal of the short lived "socio-economic" clause that recognized socio-economic conditions of the mother as a ground for approval of an interruption of pregnancy.[92]

A review of the coalition agreements entered into between the *Likud* and its coalition partners in the current government, and specifically the April 1, 2009, agreement with the *Haredi* (ultra-Orthodox) *United Torah Judaism* party,[93] has not indicated any condition regarding changing the status quo on abortions in Israel. This coalition agreement did, however, require the Ministry of Health to be headed by a Deputy Minister of Health from the *United Torah Judaism* party that would directly report to Prime Minister Binyamin Netanyahu. Mr. Yakov Litzman[94] of *United Torah Judaism* currently serves in that role.

In her 2009 article, cited above, Dr. Hashiloni-Dolev warned that the change proposed by the 2009 bill's drafters intended to provide Israeli women "full autonomy and promote their personal freedoms might awake religious bodies that until that time had closed their eyes regarding the silent agreement between the Ministry of Health and Israeli women that undergo abortions even if they do not meet the criteria in the law."[95]

She further argued that the Israeli abortion law, much like other laws in Israel, was a product of a political compromise that encouraged women to lie to the CIPs or expose before them intimate facts about their lives. According to Dr. Hashiloni-Dolev, although such an arrangement was contradictory to any feminist agenda that would negate any involvement of the state in a woman's choice, this arrangement was acceptable because in practice it enabled the approval of 98% of all requests for abortions in 2008. She therefore warned:

---

[90] *Id.*

[91] Abolition of CIPs (Amendments) Bill, 5771-2010, THE KNESSET WEBSITE, http://www.knesset.gov.il/privatelaw/data/18/2666.rtf (last visited Jan. 31, 2012)

[92] Hashiloni-Dolev, *supra* note 86.

[93] *Coalition Agreement between the Likud and United Torah Judaism Political Parties*, KNESSET (Apr. 1, 2009), http://www.knesset.gov.il/docs/heb/addCoalition2009_2.pdf.

[94] *Current Knesset Members*, THE KNESSET WEBSITE, http://www.knesset.gov.il/mk/eng/mk_eng.asp?mk_individual_id_t=216 (last visited Jan. 31, 2012).

[95] Hashiloni-Dolev, *supra* note 86.

[W]hen Knesset members pursue justice, they would better be careful not to awake demons that may at the end reach a contrary outcome. It is hoped this worry will be proven wrong and we will realize that we are ready for a law that respects the right of the woman in her body without intervention and supervision of the State of the intimate world of women.[96]

The impact of the bills submitted by liberal members of the Knesset regarding removal of restrictions to abortions on reigniting the abortion debate in Israel is unclear. A review of bills calling for the opposite result, namely for further restricting access to abortion, has identified a bill submitted by Knesset Member Nisim Zeev,[97] of the *Shas* (Sepharadi Guardians of the Torah) religious party on July 11, 2011.[98] This bill includes provisions similar to those proposed in a 2007 bill for outlawing abortions after the twenty-second week of pregnancy[99] that was rejected by the Ministerial Committee on November 8, 2010.[100]

D. Religious Leaders

In December 2010, Israel's Chief Rabbis Yona Metzger and Shlomo Amar called on all Israeli rabbis to fight what they called the "abortion epidemic in our country."[101] The Chief Rabbis, one Ashkenazi (of European descent) and the second Sephardic (of North African descent) are employed by the State and appointed in accordance with the Chief Rabbinate in Israel Law, 5740-1980.[102]

The Chief Rabbis reportedly sent a letter to rabbis all across Israel last year instructing them to "bring up the Exodus Torah reading during their sermon on Saturday regarding the 'biblical prohibition to kill fetuses in their mothers' intestines.'"[103]

The Israeli media has reported that the Rabbis' recent letters were based on the findings of a special committee appointed by the Chief Rabbinate of Israel three years ago to investigate the status of abortions in Israel. The committee found that out of the approximately 50,000 abortions allegedly carried out in Israel every year, 30,000 were illegal. Based on these findings, the Chief Rabbis have continued to stress the importance of opposing abortions every year in

---

[96] *Id.*

[97] *Knesset Member Nisim Zeev*, THE KNESSET WEBSITE, http://www.knesset.gov.il/mk/eng/mk_eng.asp?mk_individual_id_t=206 (last visited Jan. 31, 2012).

[98] SHAS HOMEPAGE, http://www.shasnet.org.il/Front/NewsNet/newspaper.asp (last visited Jan. 31, 2012).

[99] Penal Law (Provisions Regarding Interruption of Pregnancies) Bill (5768-2007) (Dec. 24, 2007), THE KNESSET WEBSITE, http://www.knesset.gov.il/privatelaw/data/17/3204.rtf; *and* (5771-2001) (July 11, 2011), *id.* at http://www.knesset.gov.il/privatelaw/data/18/3394.rtf.

[100] *The Abortion Bill Failed, Litzman Scolded His Office Employee*, YNET (Nov. 8, 2011), http://www.ynet.co.il/articles/0,7340,L-3981334,00.html.

[101] Rabbi Levi Brackman & Rivkah Lubitch, *Chief Rabbis: Fight 'Abortion Epidemic,'* YNET (Dec. 22, 2010), http://www.ynetnews.com/articles/0,7340,L-4002145,00.html.

[102] Chief Rabbinate in Israel Law, 5740-1980, 34 LSI 97 (5740-1979/89).

[103] Brackman & Lubitch, *supra* note 101.

preparation for the Exodus sermon, which talks about Hebrew midwives in Egypt who did not listen to Pharaoh's ruling and refused to cast away the male babies to the Nile.[104]

Considering abortions to be the "actual murder of souls," and noting that "[a]side from the severity of the sin, it also delays salvation,"[105] the Chief Rabbis' letter reportedly presents a three-stage plan to decrease the number of abortions in Israel:

> Firstly, the chief rabbis asked that with the help of their sermons and channels of information, the local rabbis encourage birth among the Jewish people and prevent unnecessary abortions. Secondly, they asked that the rabbis hand out pamphlets "in preparation of a happy marriage" to any couple who is to be wed. And thirdly, consult with a doctor regarding such activity.[106]

E. Political Parties' Abortion Agenda

In his weekly sermon in December 2010, *Shas'* spiritual leader Rabbi Ovadia Yosef addressed what he called the abortion "epidemic" in Israel.[107] *Shas* (abbreviation of Sepharadi Guardians of the Torah) is a political party that represents religious Israelis mainly of North African Jewish descent. Rabbi Ovadiah Yosef is a renowned *halakhic* authority and *Shas* spiritual leader.[108]

Shas's opposition to abortions was met with strong disagreement in a 2010 debate at the Knesset Committee on the Status of Woman. Knesset Member Nitzan Horowitz of the leftist party *Meretz* strongly attacked the Chief Rabbinates' actions against abortions and emphasized that women are the only ones who may make decisions on whether or not to undergo an abortion. He rejected all threats and efforts to influence women's decisions in this area.[109]

V. Religious, Cultural, and Social Norms Regarding Reproductive Care

A. Jewish Religion and Culture

It has been noted that "Jewish Israelis of all ethnic and class identities are highly family-oriented."[110] They tend to marry young, have more children, and divorce less frequently than

---

[104] *Id.*

[105] *Id.*

[106] *Id.*

[107] Kobi Nahshoni, *Rabbi Yosef: Doctors Kill the Living*, YNET (Dec. 27, 2010), http://www.ynetnews.com/articles/0,7340,L-4004368,00.html.

[108] For more information, *see* the *Shas* website, SHASNET.ORG, http://www.shasnet.org.il/Front/NewsNet/newspaper.asp (in Hebrew; last visited Feb. 1, 2012).

[109] *A Fierce Debate in the Knesset Regarding Rabbinate Activities Against Abortions*, MERETZ (Jan. 12, 2010), http://www.myparty.org.il/aspx/article.aspx?id=618 (in Hebrew).

[110] Daphna Birenbaum, *'Cheaper Than a Newcomer': On the Social Production of IVF Policy in Israel*, 26(7) SOCIOLOGY OF HEALTH & ILLNESS 897-924 (2004), *available at* http://onlinelibrary.wiley.com/doi/10.1111/j.0141-9889.2004.00422.x/pdf.

North Americans and Western Europeans. The "supreme significance of the family and child bearing for Jewish Israelis" is related to various religious, historical, cultural, social, and geopolitical conditions.[111]

> Israelis' pro-natalist attitude has been said to be

>> underpinned by major biblical texts. Jewish national identity is founded on family myths (e.g. the Patriarchs and Matriarchs). And the biblical commandment "be fruitful and multiply" constitutes childbearing as not only a goal in one's own life, but as a contribution to a collective mission.... Although at present the majority of Israeli Jews do not define themselves as "observant" and do not adhere to religious dictates, all are well acquainted with these biblical notions, which are repeatedly taught and alluded to in the national school curriculum. Thus, even for many secular Israelis, childbearing often carries the broader significance of linking oneself to the communal Jewish body.[112]

A leading 1996 Supreme Court decision reflects the Israeli cultural approach to parenthood as a basic human right. In a special procedure involving an additional hearing by a bench of eleven justices, the Court recognized that a woman's right to motherhood (by implanting her frozen ova, which had been previously fertilized with her estranged husband's semen, in a surrogate) was superior to the right of her estranged husband's not to be a father. The husband had been living with another woman and had fathered a daughter from that union. The petitioner objected to being divorced from him and requested to continue with the implantation of the fertilized ova regardless of their separation.[113] Among various considerations, the justices analyzed the contractual obligations between the spouses as well as relevant ethical and justice principles applicable in the case. They further made various references to foreign law, as well as to Jewish law and tradition.[114]

In reaching the conclusion that the wife's interest in motherhood in that case surpassed the contrary interest of the husband not to become a father, some justices in the majority referred to the high regard the Jewish culture allocates to the right to life. Justice Turkel stated, for example, that the right to be a parent must be viewed as either part of or as complimentary to the right to life. In his opinion, the right to parenthood deserves recognition as a basic independent human right and not as a derivative of freedom of choice.[115]

Consenting, Justice Tal cited God's blessing to men in Genesis to "be fruitful and multiply,"[116] as well as Sarah's (the matriarch's) desperate call to be able to bear a child.[117]

---

[111] *Id.* at 901.

[112] *Id.*

[113] For a divorce to be valid under Jewish law, both parties must consent.

[114] Additional Hearing 2401/95 Nachmani v. Nachmani, 50(4) PISKE DIN [PD] (Supreme Court Decisions) 661 (5756/57-1996).

[115] *Id.* at 736 (Turkel, J.).

[116] *Id.* (Tal, J., consenting) (quoting Genesis A, 28(8)).

[117] *Id.* at 702.

Justice Tal further cited additional sources in support of recognizing the right to bear children as "one of the most superior values" in the Jewish tradition.[118]

B. Impact of the Holocaust and Threats to State Survival

Experts have also noted the impact of the Jewish history of persecution and particularly of the Holocaust as an additional explanation for Israel's pro-natalist approach. The genocide perpetrated on Jews in the Holocaust and the ongoing loss of life in terrorist attacks and in wars since the establishment of the State are considered by some experts as having strengthened Israel's resolve to survive as a Jewish homeland in an area that is often viewed as hostile. This resolve seems to be directly connected with Israel's public policy in support of reproductive rights.[119]

VI. Medical Reproductive Care Providers and Barriers to Care

Reproductive care is provided by authorized medical centers, both public and private. In 2007 there were twenty-three medical centers that provided IVF care. Abortions must similarly be performed by authorized medical centers, as discussed earlier in this report. Specific legal requirements apply to all medical service providers in Israel—physicians, nurses, and others. Barriers to care have also been discussed earlier in this report. They generally apply in cases where the circumstances do not meet the criteria established by law.

NGOs are generally not authorized to perform any medical procedures. Some NGOs, however, are active in providing information regarding reproductive rights and in trying to impact Israeli public opinion either directly or through lobbing the Knesset (Parliament).

The main pro-life organization in Israel is *Efrat*; their objective is "to increase the Jewish birthrate in Israel."[120] The organization lobbies against abortions and offers financial support for women to continue their pregnancies. *Efrat* is registered as a nonprofit organization in accordance with Israeli law. Another organization that provides financial support and counseling to pregnant women in Israel is Just One Life (JOL),[121] in Hebrew is known as *Nefesh Achat B'Yisrael*. JOL appears to be a U.S.-based organization, as its website declares that it is a "501(c)(3) nonprofit organization."[122]

---

[118] *Id.* at 702-03.

[119] For an in-depth analysis of the elements impacting Israel's pro-natalist policy, *see* Daniel Sperling, *Commanding the "Be Fruitful and Multiply" Directive: Reproductive Ethics, Law, and Policy in Israel*, 19 CAMBRIDGE Q. 363-71 (2010); *and* Daniel Sperling & Yael Simon, *Attitudes and Policies Regarding Access to Fertility Care and Assisted Reproductive Technologies in Israel*, 21 REPRODUCTIVE BIOMEDICINE ONLINE 854-61 (2010).

[120] For more information, *see About Us*, EFRAT, http://www.efrat.org.il/english/about/default.asp (last visited Jan. 31, 2012).

[121] JUST 1 LIFE, http://www.justonelife.org/about.asp (last visited Jan. 31, 2012).

[122] *Id.*

There are several NGOs that provide information to Israelis wishing to bear children. For example, the Hen Association for Fertility and Life website states that the association's objective is to assist couples who suffer from infertility.[123] The association provides general information on relevant laws and reproductive services.

VII. Government Funding for Reproductive Care

A. Funding Policy for Reproductive Care

Israel has allocated funding for various types of reproductive care. Both legal abortions[124] and ART (Assisted Reproductive Technology) treatments (including fertility treatments in which both eggs and sperm are handled in the laboratory, and IVF and related procedures)[125] are included in such care. An author has commented:

> The United States and Israel are widely regarded as possessing two of the most ART … friendly environments in the world. Both countries stand at the epicenter of fertility-related research and practice and support the supply and demand sides of the ART market with avidity.[126]

The two countries' policies, however, are in sharp contrast with regard to public financing of ART. In "stark contrast to the United States," Israel has invested heavily "in providing wide and free access to ART treatment as part of 'the basic package of health benefits guaranteed by the Government.'"[127]

B. Types of Public Funding of Reproductive Care

The Knesset passed a National Health Insurance Law in June 1994.[128] Pursuant to that Law, Israeli residents are insured by registered health funds of their choice. In addition to premiums paid by members, the health funds receive government subsidies in correlation to their membership size.

Appendix 2 of the Law lists various tests and services that must be covered by the health funds (hereafter "Health Services Basket"). Among those services, the appendix lists the following types of covered services for reproductive care:

---

[123] HEN ASSOCIATION FOR FERTILITY AND LIFE, http://www.amotatchen.org/ (in Hebrew; last visited Jan. 31, 2012).

[124] *See* Part III of this report.

[125] Definition of reproductive care provided by Ellen Waldmann, *Cultural Priorities Revealed: The Development and Regulation of Assisted Reproduction in the United States and Israel*, 16 HEALTH MATRIX 65, 67 (2006), *cited in* Guy I. Seidman, *Regulating Life and Death: The Case of Israel's "Health Basket" Committee*, 23 J. CONTEMP. HEALTH & POL'Y 9, 52 n.174 (2006-2007).

[126] Seidman, *supra* note 125, at 52.

[127] *Id*. at 54.

[128] National Health Insurance Law, SH 5754, p. 156, *as amended*.

1. *Tests*

– Lab: fetal protein;[129]

– Endocrinology: sex hormones;[130] and

– Fertility tests, including[131]

- numeric diagnosis of semen;
- numeric and qualitative diagnosis of semen cell movement;
- morphologic diagnosis of semen cells including electronic microscopic diagnosis;
- comprehensive bacteriologic test for presence of microorganisms in urine, urine flow, and discharge of prostate;
- various biochemical and enzymatic tests that reflect proper activity of the male glands; and
- tests for detecting woman's infertility, including tests for the need for in vitro fertilization (IVF).

2. *Fertility Treatments*

– Diagnosis and treatment of infertility, including treatments for improvement of semen and hormonal treatments; and

– IVF treatments for the purpose of the birth of two children for couples who do not have children from their present marriage, as well as for childless women who wish to establish a single-parent family.[132]

Eligibility for fertility treatments varies depending on the Health Fund to which the patient subscribes. For example, different health funds have different limitations on the number and frequency of treatments. Similarly, differences may also exist regarding eligibility for fertility-related medications, although certain medications are listed in the Health Services Basket to which all patients are entitled, subject to deductibles. In 2011, treatments designed to preserve the fertility of women who are expected to undergo chemotherapy or radiation treatments through the preservation of ova, fetuses, and umbilical cords were added to the treatments that are included in the Health Services Basket.[133]

The State subsidizes PGD (Pre-implantation Genetic Diagnosis) in cases involving certain diseases.[134] Although the State does not subsidize ova donations, it covers all expenses related to an IVF treatment that involves ova donations.[135]

---

[129] *Id.* 2d App., § 3A(11).

[130] *Id.* § 3C(5).

[131] *Id.* § 3G.

[132] *Id.* § 6D.

[133] Expansion of the Basket of Health Services for 2011, Directive No. 6/2011 (Jan. 23, 2011), MINISTRY OF HEALTH, http://www.health.gov.il/hozer/mr06_2011.pdf (in Hebrew; last visited Jan. 31, 2012).

[134] Memorandum issued by KIRC, *supra* note 5.

3. *Genetic Testing*

The State subsidizes genetic testing for the following diseases: Tay-Sachs (TSD), cystic fibrosis, thalassemia, and Familial Dysautonomia (FD).[136]

4. *Services During Pregnancy*

Services that must be covered by insurance during pregnancy include visits to doctors and nurses of the expectant mother's health fund, standard blood tests, glucose tolerance tests, one fetal system test, high-risk hospitalization, and birth in a hospital.[137]

5. *Interruption of Pregnancy*

Abortions that are approved by the State are free for all girls younger than nineteen years of age and in some other circumstances.[138]

C. Funding Amounts for Reproductive Care

Based on information received from the Knesset Information and Research Center (KIRC) in 2011, the total amount allocated by the Ministry of Health for services that were included in the basket of health services for the State's over 7.7 million residents[139] was estimated as NIS 31 billions (about US$8.29 billion).[140] Of that amount, different budget allocations were made by the different Health Funds for reproductive care services.[141]

According to KIRC, information regarding the total budget spent on reproductive care services in Israel was unavailable at the Ministry of Health as of March 2011, the date of the KIRC Memorandum. According to KIRC's calculations and estimates based on a collection of

---

[135] *Id.* at 2.

[136] *Addition to the Health Services Basket, Screening Tests for Couples With Family Likelihood of Bearing Children with Familial Dysautonomia FD*, MINISTRY OF HEALTH (Nov. 4, 2008), http://www.health.gov.il/ download/forms/a3243_mr41_08.pdf (in Hebrew); *see also Department for Locality Medicine Information*, MINISTRY OF HEALTH, http://www.health.gov.il/pages/default.asp?PageId=1696&catId=217&maincat=42 (last updated Jan. 24, 2011).

[137] *Tests During Pregnancy*, DEPARTMENT FOR THE MOTHER, THE CHILD, AND YOUTH, MINISTRY OF HEALTH, http://www.health.gov.il/pages/default.asp?pageid=866&parentid=854&catid=116&maincat=35 (in Hebrew; last visited Jan. 12, 2011).

[138] *Expansion of Eligibility for Interruption of Pregnancy for Teens under Nineteen Years of Age, Directive No. 38/2008, supra* note 77 and further discussion in Part III, above.

[139] *Press Release: 63rd Independence Day – Approximately 7,746,000 Residents in the State of Israel*, ISRAEL CENTRAL BUREAU OF STATISTICS (May 8, 2011), http://www1.cbs.gov.il/www/hodaot2011n/ 11_11_101e.pdf.

[140] Memorandum issued by KIRC, *supra* note 5,.at 1.

[141] *See* Part II(A) of this report, "Prenatal Care Insurance Coverage," for an explanation of health insurance services through Health Funds.

reports from the different Health Funds in response to the author's request, the total amount spent by Israeli Health Funds on fertility, pregnancy, and delivery services in 2010 was NIS 529 million (about $US140 million), in addition to NIS 1.7 billion (about $US4.5 million) paid by the Institute of Social Security (ISC) to hospitals for delivery fees.[142]

According to KIRC, considering the total budget allocated for health services in 2010, Health Funds' spending on all reproductive services formed 1.76% of the total basket of services budget.[143]

1. Fertility Treatments

Most of the expense for fertility treatment relates to IVF procedures. In 2010 it was estimated that Israeli Health Funds spent NIS 407 million (about $US109 million) in this area. This may not include some medications that are not classified as fertility medications but are prescribed during fertility treatments.[144]

2. Pregnancy and Delivery

In 2010 it was estimated that Israeli Health Funds spent NIS 108 million (about US$28.84 million) for pregnancy and delivery services. In addition, the State, through the Institute for Social Security (ISC), transfers to hospitals fees for delivery services performed by them. According to KIRC, in 2009 ISC transferred NIS 1.7 billion (about US$454 million), and a slightly higher amount was transferred in 2010.[145]

3. Interruption of Pregnancy

In 2010 the Health Funds paid NIS 14 million (about US$3.74 million) for services related to abortions.[146]

VIII. Women's Health Care and Reproductive Policy: The Stakeholders

In general, the stakeholders in women's health care and reproductive policy outcomes potentially include the following:

- Pharmaceutical companies;
- Medical device companies;
- Medical researchers;

---

[142] Memorandum issued by KIRC, *supra* note 5, at 4.

[143] *Id.*

[144] *Id.*

[145] *Id.*

[146] *Id.*

- Physicians' groups;

- Patients' groups;

- Health Funds (medical insurance companies); and

- The State

IX. Reproductive Policy Advocacy

There are various PACs and NGOs that act in an effort to promote opposing views on reproductive policy in Israel.

The Joint Action Committee (a 501(c)(4) organization), for example, is a U.S. advocacy group that declares its objective as the promotion of both U.S.-Israel relations and what it describes as "reproductive freedom, separation of religion and state, and social policies in keeping with the core values of the American Jewish community."[147]

Pro-life, Israeli-based organizations, such as *Efrat* and *Be-ad Chaim* (For Life) are registered as nonprofit organizations (*Amutot*) in Israel. *Efrat* has announced that it has solicited support from U.S. Members of Congress.[148]

X. Impact of Neighboring Countries' Laws and Policies on Israel's Reproductive Policies

Israel's population, the majority of which is Jewish, was estimated in May 2011 at nearly 7.75 million.[149] Israel is surrounded by Arab Muslim states with relatively high fertility rates. "According to the revised population estimates of the United Nations, the population of Arab countries rose from 171.6 million in 1980 to 300.2 million in 2002."[150]

Although Israel's population (and geographical size) is extremely minute as compared with that of the twenty-two Arab states in the region, regional demographic concerns, where they exist, have generally focused on the fertility rates of Arab-Israelis and of Palestinians, and not on neighboring countries' reproductive policies and laws.[151]

---

[147] For more information, *see About JAC*, JOINT ACTION COMMITTEE, http://www.jacpac.org/index. php/who-we-are/about-us (last visited Jan. 31, 2012).

[148] *See Efrat holds Luncheon on Capitol Hill*, YESHIVA WORLD NEWS, http://www.theyeshivaworld. com/article.php?p=6517 (last visited Jan. 31, 2012).

[149] *Press Release: 63rd Independence Day – Approximately 7,746,000 Residents in the State of Israel*, ISRAEL CENTRAL BUREAU OF STATISTICS, *supra* note 139.

[150] UN ECONOMIC AND SOCIAL COMMISSION FOR WESTERN ASIA (ESCWA), THE DEMOGRAPHIC PROFILE OF ARAB COUNTRIES, AGING OF RURAL POPULATIONS 2 (Dec. 31, 2007), *available at* http://www.globalaging. org/ruralaging/world/2008/arabrural.pdf.

[151] *See, e.g., Demographic Trends in the Land of Israel (1800–2007)*, THE INSTITUTE FOR ZIONIST STRATEGIES, http://www.izs.org.il/eng/default.asp?father_id=114&catid=118&itemid=208 (last visited Jan. 31, 2012).

In analyzing Israel's pro-natalist policy, one social welfare and health scholar has noted that practitioners and activists who have argued over the years for increased funding for IVF and ART have repeatedly tied the need to support such procedures to demographic concerns. She quoted two statements by Knesset members specifically connecting IVF funding to the increasing Jewish population in Israel.[152]

Although demographic concerns may have contributed to Israel's pro-natalist policies, this report has discussed how these policies have been more affected by general, pro-natalist cultural attitudes, along with the historic threat to Jewish survival culminating in the Holocaust. These attitudes, as discussed earlier in this report, appear to have played a stronger role in shaping state policies on reproductive rights.

Prepared by Ruth Levush
Senior Foreign Law Specialist
February 2012

---

[152] Birenbaum, *supra* note 110, at 905.

www.ingramcontent.com/pod-product-compliance
Lightning Source LLC
Chambersburg PA
CBHW080623180526
45168CB00007B/3033